Protein

Protein Food

By Cathy Wilson
Copyright © 2014

Income Disclaimer

This book contains business strategies, marketing methods and other business advice that, regardless of my own results and experience, may not produce the same results (or any results) for you. I make absolutely no guarantee, expressed or implied, that by following the advice below you will make any money or improve current profits, as there are several factors and variables that come into play regarding any given business.

Primarily, results will depend on the nature of the product or business model, the conditions of the marketplace, the experience of the individual, and situations and elements that are beyond your control.
As with any business endeavor, you assume all risk related to investment and money based on your own discretion and at your own potential expense.

Liability Disclaimer
By reading this book, you assume all risks associated with using the advice given below, with a full understanding that you, solely, are responsible for anything that may occur as a result of putting this information into action in any way, and regardless of your interpretation of the advice.
You further agree that our company cannot be held responsible in any way for the success or failure of your business as a result of the information presented in this book. It is your responsibility to conduct your own due diligence regarding the safe and successful operation of your business if you intend to apply any of our information in any way to your business operations.

Terms of Use
You are given a non-transferable, "personal use" license to this book. You cannot distribute it or share it with other individuals.

Also, there are no resale rights or private label rights granted when purchasing this book. In other words, it's for your own personal use only.

Protein

Protein Food

By Cathy Wilson

Table of Contents

6

Introduction

If you want to keep your cells healthy, grow and develop opti-mally, and build lean muscle to blast pesky fat, you've gotta eat protein, according to nutrition experts at *Medline Plus!*

This introductory guide gives you all the basic information you need to know about protein, in order to build your healthy eating plan for life. The focus is to understand how important protein is in your overall health and wellness.

Think of this guide as a pocketbook of information. Something you can use as a reference tool to strengthen your overall health and wellness betterment knowledge.

FACT - Without protein on a routine basis, you wouldn't survive very long.

Protein is one of three macronutrients your body requires to function. A macronutrient just means you need this nutrient in large amounts. Protein isn't something your body manufactures internally, which means you've got to get it from a food source daily. You can't store protein for long periods of time, so eating it regularly is important.

This essential nutrient comes in different types; complete and incomplete. In this book you'll learn the difference, and gather the knowledge required to ensure you're getting the best protein for you, considerate of your preferences and tolerances.

Protein is a food factor that can help you lose weight and sustain it. Time for you to learn how!

Chapter One - What is Protein?

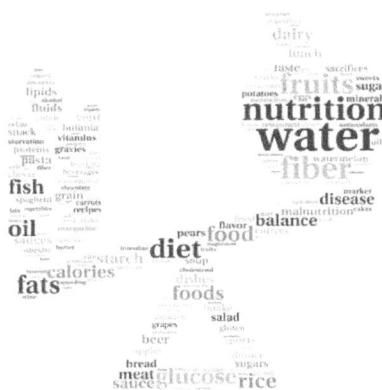

Medical News Today says, proteins are large molecules that have specific amino acids which your body and the cells in your body requires to function optimally. Your body cells, structure, cell regulation, function, tissues and organs, can't survive without protein. Protein is also responsible for transporting oxygen to your internal systems via your blood, acting as a neurotransmitter.

*Every cell in your body has protein! That's how important this macronutrient is.

FACT - About 20 percent of your body is protein.

All your body tissues; skin, organs, muscles and bones contain protein.

Pseudonyms - Did you know that antibodies, hormones and enzymes are proteins?

According to *Iowa State University Nutrition Department*, there's over 10,000 different proteins required to maintain your good health.

Protein is made of amino acids, which are the building blocks of life. They're adhered together in various patterns to create specific proteins, for slightly different function. There are 20 amino acids in total. Eight of these are essential, which means your body can't make them, so you've got to get them by eating.

These amino acids circulate constantly throughout your bloodstream and are used when required, or consumed to make protein.

As mentioned previously, the two main types of protein are complete and incomplete.

COMPLETE PROTEIN

Fitday states, a complete protein must have all 20 amino acids present in the food. Animal and fish foods are your best option to get complete protein. Beef, chicken, milk, and yogurt, are examples of compete protein sources.

INCOMPLETE PROTEIN

These are protein sources that lack one or more of the 20 essential amino acids. Many people call these partial proteins. I think of this as you might a puzzle. In order to form a complete protein you're going to need the right combination of partial proteins, in the right amounts. That's where it gets a tad tricky.

Most plant source proteins are incomplete. The exception is quinoa, which is a grain complete protein source.

Vegetarians often have a protein deficiency, simply because they may be eating protein-rich plant sources, but if they are missing any one of the essential amino acids, their body doesn't have the recipe to create protein for use. Whole grain, beans, peas and seeds, are typical incomplete protein sources.

Essential Amino Acids

The 8 EEA you've got to eat each day for optimal health are; valine, tyrosine, leucine, isoleucine, methionine, phenylalanine, lysine, and tryptophan.

Valine - Necessary for muscle development.

Tyrosine - An antioxidant that helps with alertness. A precursor of adrenaline, norepinephrine, and dopamine.

Leucine - Helps promote growth hormone synthesis. Important for speeding up wound healing, and healthy skin and hair.

Isoleucine - Important for red blood cell formation.

Methionine - This antioxidant helps break down fats for use, and interferes with muscle breakdown.

Phenylalanine - Aids in sharpening your memory and maintaining a healthy nervous system.

Lysine - Important for optimal nervous system function. Also essential part of muscle protein, and the creation of hormones and enzymes.

Tryptophan - Aids in relieving head pain and is important in the creation of the neurotransmitter serotonin.

Non-Essential Amino Acids

These AA are produced by your body as long as you supply adequate amounts of carbon, oxygen, hydrogen, and nitrogen in your diet. The non-essential amino acids are; alanine, cysteine, glycine, serine, histidine, taurine, cysteine, proline, asparagine, aspartic acid, glutathione, and glutamine.

Alanine - Helps remove toxins from muscle breakdown.

Cysteine - An antioxidant found in abundance in the protein of skin, hair, and nails.

Glycine - A neurotransmitter helpful in wound healing.

Serine - Great for muscle growth.

Histidine - Helps improve blood flow and feeling sexy. Also critical for synthesis of red and white blood cells.

Taurine - Helps with optimal brain function.

Cysteine - Helps remove toxins and make skin.

Proline - Important for inter-cell communication.

Asparagine - Assists in balancing your emotions.

Aspartic Acid - Important for immune system protein synthesis and removing ammonia and other harmful toxins from your body.

Glutathione - Helps remove toxins and fights aging.

Glutamine - Important for the synthesis of genetic molecules.

How Much Protein does your Body Need?

14

According to nutrition experts, the recommended protein intake for the average American is .4 grams per pound per day, if you want to get technical. More if you are training hard. To keep it simple, we're going to go with 2-3 servings per day. Which translates to about 40-60 grams, where a typical 3-4 ounce serving of complete protein is about 20 grams of protein. That's just to give you an ideal.

We often get into trouble figuring out what constitutes a serving. If you're conditioned to expect restaurant portions, I can guarantee you're in for a gynormous shock. Typical restaurant portions are 3-4 times larger than the average person requires for optimal health.

Protein Serving Size

*3-4 ounces per serving, where 1 ounce has about 7 grams of protein

*1-2 tbsp. peanut butter

*1 cup skim milk

*Piece of chicken or steak about the size of a deck of cards

*2x2 inch cube of cheese

These are typical examples of complete protein, and the serving size your body requires to get adequate protein. Complete protein is the optimal choice because it's easily absorbed and you know there aren't any amino acids missing. If there are, the food is not considered a complete protein and can't be used as such.

CIP - Cathy's Important Point - If you're training hard, you'll want to increase your lean complete protein intake. Particularly just prior to and after a workout. This gives your body a chance to breakdown and rebuild your muscle bigger and stronger.

NOTE - A muscular body burns more calories at rest that a fatty one of the same weight. Muscle weighs more than fat, is smaller, more aesthetically pleasing, provides energy, deters injury, and naturally boosts your metabolism to help keep fat gone for good!

My Thoughts...

Protein is one of those nutrients that's definitely been around the block a few times. A few years back, the media seemed to steer people away from protein, convincing the general populous that protein made you grow big muscles and get fat. Which of course is completely absurd!

In fact the opposite is true. By eating lean complete protein in the right amounts, you'll build lean muscle mass, which boost your metabolism and helps you blast fat.

A happy note for you as we move on to learn more.

Chapter Two - Protein Benefits

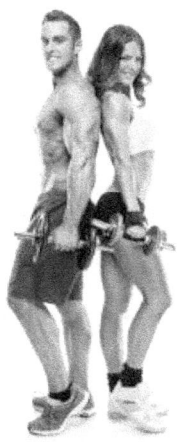

As with everything in life, finding the right balance is the priority. You need protein to be healthy, and too little or too much creates a negative.

Here are the benefits of getting just the right amount of protein in your daily diet!

*MORE MUSCLE - LEANER BODY

Protein stimulates protein synthesis and helps deter immediate protein breakdown, which helps sustain and build lean protein muscle mass. Eating protein helps ensure your body doesn't lose or start breaking down protein for energy, and promotes muscle strength and development.

*INCREASED METABOLISM

Muscle burns more calories than fat. And when you're getting adequate protein and building lean muscle, your body's' naturally working harder for you. Using more energy to blast fat and get you super skinny strong!

*EAT LESS

Poliquingroup health experts report, eating less triggers your thermic effect. Where the food and protein requires almost twice the calories to breakdown carbs. Take note that fat requires the least amount of energy to metabolize all three. In other words, protein fills you up with energy that lasts longer, and it works harder for you burning off more energy.

*FASTER MUSCLE BUILDING

Research studies show that fueling your body with adequate complete protein aides in faster muscle building. Fueling your body with protein before and immediately after a workout is essential in preventing the breakdown of muscles to be used for energy.

If you don't get enough protein in your diet, your body will naturally start breaking down from the inside out. Your muscles will be taken apart, and this protein will be used to give your body energy. Talk about defeating the purpose of training hard to get thin and muscular sexy!

*LESS TUMMY FAT

Experts from *Nutrition Daily* state that quality complete protein at every meal encourages belly fat shrinkage. Scientists believe about 10 grams per meal is the minimum protein required to trigger protein synthesis and fat burn.

*IMPROVED STRENGTH

Oodles of studies show that a diet with adequate protein encourages a stronger body. Makes sense because muscle strength is a factor in overall body strength. Eat your protein to build your muscles bigger and stronger, and you're going to continue to build your overall body strength.

*LESS INJURY AND FASTER RECOVERY

A lean muscular body decreases the risk of injury and reduces recovery time when an injury occurs. *Dr. Mirkin* reports, eating protein immediately after an intense training session helps you recover faster.

If you want to improve your strength, endurance, and speed, you've gotta exercise hard enough to injure your muscles. So when you're muscles heal, they're stronger. That's how you build muscle. You work hard and damage it, eat your protein and build it stronger.

*IMPROVED THINKING

Protein is involved in energy production, hunger, motivation, thinking, and wakefulness. Scientific research shows that various brain disorders like ADHD and schizophrenia, are associated with inadequate absorption of protein.

Protein is a brain food, so make sure you eat a diverse range of protein daily if you want to think clearly.

*BETTER QUALITY SLEEP

Research shows that protein is somehow interconnected with your internal sleep - wake cycle. Protein may optimize chemical transmitter balance, helping you to settle down to sleep at night, and trigger you energized to battle your day.

It's also important to note that complex healthy carbs just before bed may actually help you get to sleep, because they trigger the release or serotonin, your sleep drug. However, it's the protein that's going to help you stay asleep. So it's important for you to find your healthy balance.

*DECREASED BLOOD PRESSURE

Health experts report, studies show lower blood pressure in individuals suffering from hypertension, when protein intake is increased. This could be from the natural increase in calorie burn associated with eating healthy protein in the right amounts.

*LONGER LIFE

Having a healthy strong mind and body is associated with living longer. By focusing on quality protein and removing simple carbs from your diet, you'll help to level blood sugars, reduce your risk of diabetes and cancers, and ward or cardiovascular disease.

In particular, a diet high in whey protein is proven to increase longevity by elevating the most powerful antioxidant we have, which is glutathione. Individuals with higher levels of this antioxidant decrease their risk of disease and dying.

Smart Protein Moves

*Don't overcook protein or you'll lose nutrients.

*By eating a large volume of higher protein plant foods you'll counteract the acid content found in animal protein foods.

*Include lots of fresh fruits and veggies for added fiber in a protein rich diet. This helps remove some of the protein stress from oxidization.

*Eating at least 1.5 g or protein per kg will help minimize muscle loss when eating to lose weight.

*Eat a wide variety of protein from both animal and plant sources in order to optimize your protein intake and optimal health gain. Protein supplementation will also help balance your protein absorption goals.

My Thoughts...

Protein aids in the restocking of lost blood, body development, wound healing, hair, nail and skin growth, and the regeneration of dead cells. It's required for the smooth internal running of your body, and prevents muscle breakdown from protein energy when adequate protein energy isn't available.

For optimal health you need 2-3 servings of protein each day. Just one more important piece of the puzzle toward your optimal diet plan.

Chapter Three - Consequences Protein Symptoms and Disease

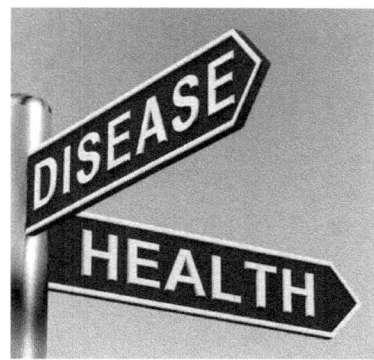

Inadequate amounts of protein can result in serious illness and disease. You need protein in order to provide your body with optimal energy to function properly. Along with building and maintaining lean muscle strength, and keeping your hair, nails, and skin healthy.

Symptoms of Protein Deficiency

Injuries that take forever to heal
Persistent head pain
Moodiness
Sudden changes in skin
Passing out
Lines across your nails
Unexplained weight loss
Mental problems in severe cases
Depression and anxiety

Extreme tiredness
Constant craving
Constipation
Apathy
Brittle nails
Hair loss
Bed sores
Tummy upset or persistent feeling of unwell
Bloated feeling
Dry and scaly skin
Sore and tired achy muscles

NOTE - If you are experiencing the above symptoms it's important to seek immediate medical attention. Better safe than sorry!

Diseases Associated With Protein Deficiency

Particularly infants and young children are vulnerable to serious growth issues with protein deficiency. Many children in third world countries die from diseases causes by inadequate protein. Makes me sad to think about the fact it's a tragic reality for many.

KWASHIORKOR

According to *Healthgrades*, Kwashiorkor is common protein deficiency in areas with drought and famine. Where there just isn't enough protein in the diet to get healthy.

Symptoms include slow growth, lethargy, swelling of the abdomen, weak immune system, skin changes, and continuous muscle loss. This disease can be prevented with adequate protein intake. However many of the effects are not reversible, as much of this occurs during the development and growth process.

MARASMUS

This is another form of severe malnutrition where muscle, tissue, and fat chronically waste away. The result of lack of protein and calories. Marasmus is the most serious PEM, or protein-energy malnutrition in the world, according to experts at *HealthGrades.*

Children are most seriously afflicted in developing nations. The problem gets worse when these children are drinking contaminated water that complicates the condition.

Symptoms include:

*Diarrhea
*Fatigue
*Fainting
*Dizziness
*Extreme weight loss

Note: Seek immediate medical attention if you're experiencing these symptoms.

CACHEXIA

Also referred to as the wasting syndrome, cachexia is the dramatic weight loss and atrophy found in patients suffering from chronic illness, including MS, diabetes, cancer, HIV, and people in a 'failure to thrive" scenario.

The weight loss is unintentional, usually associated with disease. According to *AboutHealth*, cachexia is present in at least 50% of people with advanced cancer, and causes 20% of cancer deaths. This disease causes weakened skeletal muscles and decrease in protein.

PROTEIN C AND PROTEIN S DEFICIENCY

Protein C and S are natural substances in your blood that deter your blood from clotting. Think of them as natural blood thinners. Having a deficiency in one or both of these proteins leaves you high risk for abnormal blood clot development.

This protein issue can be acquired if you lack vitamin K, or suffer from liver disease, kidney disease, or HIV.

Symptoms of Blood Clot

*Pain and swelling in a leg or arm (like a Charlie horse)
*Purple or red skin
*Warm to feel

If a blood clot or Deep Vein Thrombosis (DVT) has broken off you need to seek immediate medical attention!

Lung Clot or Pulmonary Embolism Symptoms

*Trouble breathing
*Trying to breathe and getting chest pain
*Heart palpitations
*Passing out
*Spitting up blood

My Thoughts...

Protein deficiency is often preventable if you're aware of the symptoms and take action. It's important that you look towards prevention by ensuring you're getting your 2-3 servings of complete lean protein each day.

Getting adequate amounts of health protein each day is all a part of healthy living. A responsibility that needs to be taken seriously because it's important. Your health is your number one asset. Never forget it!

Chapter Four - Protein Foods

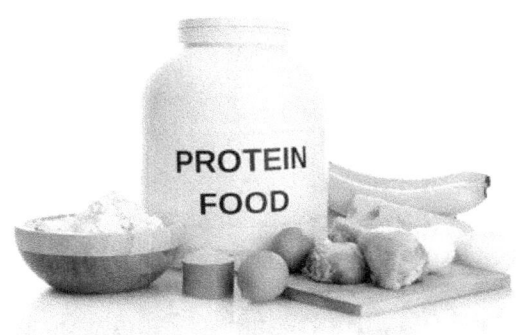

According to the *Choosemyplate* government publication, foods associated with meats, fish, poultry, seafood, eggs, legumes, peas, soy, seeds, and nuts, are all a part of the protein food group. Eating a wide variety of protein foods is your best bet to ensure adequate muscle building protein to get sexy strong.

2-3 servings is what the average adult requires. Of course this may change if you are in training, have an absorption issue, or other underlying medical condition.

Complete Protein Foods

Poultry, Meat and Fish - Fish, pork, game, beef, chicken, and turkey work. It's best to stick with leaner cuts of meat like beef tenderloin and ground round.

Dairy and Eggs - Eggs are an excellent source of complete protein. Milk, hard cheese and yogurt are also good choices. Just make sure you keep to lower-fat and moderation.

Vegan Choices - There are a few complete whole food choices of protein from plant sources including quinoa, soy milk, tofu, and edamame.

Foods Highest in Complete Protein

Chicken Breast - 50 grams - 15 grams protein

Hard Cheese - 1 ounce - 9 grams protein

Low-Fat Cottage Cheese - 1/2 cup - 13 grams protein

Salmon - 3 ounce serving - 20 grams protein

Lean Beef - 3 ounces - 30 grams protein

Pork Chops - 3-4 ounces - 30 grams protein

Soy Beans - 1/2 cup - 15 grams protein

Tofu - 3 ounces - 5 grams protein

Milk and Milk Products - 1 cup - 13 grams, 1/2 cup yogurt - 8 grams protein

Eggs - 1 egg - 5 grams protein, 2 egg whites - 10 grams protein

Seed and Nuts - 1 ounce - 8 grams protein

Incomplete Protein Foods

*Seeds and nuts

*Whole grains

*Legumes

*Veggies

Complementary Protein

These are protein sources that aren't complete and can stand alone. They don't have to be eaten at the same sitting, just sometime during the same day, according to *Natural Medicine.*

Food Pairings that Make Complete Protein

Legumes and nuts/seeds with dairy

Dairy with grains

Legumes with nuts

Legumes with dairy

Legumes with grains

Legumes with seeds

Dairy with nuts

Common Foods That Complement Each Other's Protein

Nuts and yogurt

Black bean salad with quinoa and cheese

Pizza

*Lasagna

*Tacos with beans

*Peanut butter sandwich on whole grain bread

*Pasta and cheese

*Rice with beans

*Chicken stir-fry

*Whole grain crackers and hummus

My Thoughts...

Balance is what you're looking for. Understanding the type of protein you should be eating is just as important as getting the right amounts.

A wise-owl move is to always choose a diverse range of protein sources, both complete and incomplete, in your diet daily. This way you can tune into what your body is saying to see if you're hitting the mark with protein!

Chapter 5- Tips to get More Protein into Your Diet

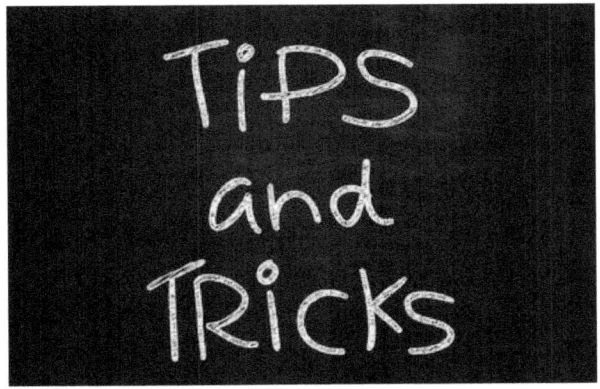

Unfortunately WAY too many people get too much of the wrong kind of protein. Just think fried fast-food crap and you're on the right track. But still, there are many of us training hard at the gym trying to build lean muscle and blast fat, and we need more protein.

One option is to down a protein shake. But they're usually disgusting and grow old fast. Here are a few *real food* moves to boost your healthy protein intake to ensure you're getting enough to fuel your body optimally.

Slip-Trick with Protein Power

Protein powder stand alone is YUK! However, if you cleverly add it to your smoothie, or slip a little into your oatmeal or muffins, it's not too bad. You may have to shop around to find one you like. I tend to stick with vanilla flavor cuz it seems to go better with everything.

Mooo-ve Into Lean Meats

We all know lean meat is an excellent source of complete protein that's easily absorbable. Add a grilled chicken break to you spinach salad. Or try some lean beef in you veggie soup. Lean cuts of meat grilled, barbecued, steamed, baked, or broiled is a wise-owl move.

Greek Yogurt

This yogurt has about half the calories and twice as much protein as normal yogurt. Better bang for your buck!

Go Fishing!

Fish is an excellent source of protein. Opt for some grilled salmon and you're getting your protective heart healthy omega fatty acids too!

Cottage Cheese Mania

People seem to either love cottage cheese or hate it. Bottom line is, cottage cheese is an excellent source of protein, with almost 15 grams in half a cup. Add some banana to it in the morning for a fantabulous energy kick. My mom used to have cottage cheese with pineapple, sprinkled with sunflower seeds for lunch all the time. Use your imagination!

Peanut Butter and Anything!

A tablespoon of peanut butter has almost 5 grams of protein. You can add peanut butter to your smoothie drink, or dip apples in it for a snack. Peanut butter can easily be added to baking, put it on your celery, or have a spoonful of it heading out the door!

Sprinkle Nuts Here, There, and Everywhere

Nuts are a fantabulous source of protein and good fat. Just re-member about 1/4 is a serving, which is about a small handful. Add nuts to dry cereal for a snack, into your stir-fry or salad, and you can even sprinkle a little on your ice-cream, or yogurt.

Just be careful you don't go overboard because they're loaded with calories.

Don't Count Out Plant-Based Protein

Just because a food source may not be a complete protein, doesn't mean it's not a healthy move for you. Make sure you add brown rice, barley, broccoli, beans, sweet potato, and spin-ach into your meal plan to optimize your total protein intake. Keep it diverse and your body will thank you for it.

Go Sushi Style

Sushi is fish, so it's a fantabulous source of protein. Don't be afraid to incorporate a sushi night into your week just to be sure you're not lacking in the lean protein department.

Go Eggy!

Adding eggs to your day is easy. Make them hardboiled to take with you. Whole grain egg wraps are another great snack be-fore working out. Add an egg or two to your smoothie, or just scramble some up! At 5 grams of protein per egg, all you've gotta to is crack a few open and you're well on your way to reaching your daily protein benchmark.

Grab a Can of Tuna

Canned tuna in water has almost 20 grams of protein and just .2 grams of fat, according to experts at *Helpguide*. Some peo-ple eat it right from the can. Or you can add it to salad, or make a sandwich. It's just an easy route to getting muscle building protein.

Whey Protein Powder

I'll be the first to admit this stuff is gross on its own. But when you toss it into your morning smoothie, pudding, or baking, you really don't even know it's there. Just 1/3 cup has almost 20 grams of protein and less than a gram of fat. Definitely something you'll wanna try.

Protein Bars

You've got to be careful here cuz many of these bars are LOADED with sugar. Take care to read the label and make sure there's at least 10 grams of protein, and the bar is less than 250 calories, with minimal sugar. You don't want to be chomping down of what might as well be a chocolate bar!

My Thoughts...

There are oodles of tips and tricks to get more protein into your day. It all starts with committing to it, and learning through trial and error what works best for you.

Take these ideas and experiment with them a little. With a little time and patience you'll find your groove and protein won't be an issue.

Chapter Six - Myths and Truths – Protein

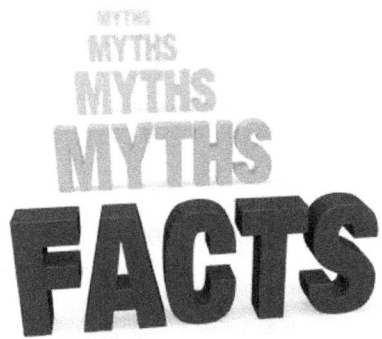

I don't care what you're talking about, there's always a black sheep that seems to distort some truths. And I'm going to knock that sheep of their rocker!

If you've got accurate information about protein, you can make better health decisions for you. That's what's important.

Time to wipeout a few protein myths once and for all.

Fallacy One - Protein powder is better than real food.

The Truth - Since when has synthetic been better than the real deal? Yes there are excellent protein powders on the market, but each person is different and what might be absorbed in one person just fine, might not work with another. The PERFECT combinations of complete proteins for protein synthesis comes from real food.

According to *Flex*, many bodybuilders report a difference in muscle building mass when they're on straight protein powder, and when they use it in combination with real complete protein foods like red meat. Consistently they don't gain as much muscle when they only use protein powders and drinks.

That's proof enough you should opt for real foods for protein, and supplement when necessary. A combination is best!

Fallacy Two - Protein requirements should stay the same.

The Truth - Whether your goal is to build muscle and lose weight, or just maintain your weight, protein intake should never stay the same. If you want continuous results with no plateaus you need to change things up in life. This includes everything from types of foods and quantity, to longer and shorter exercise programs, that vary in intensity, weights, and cardiovascular activity.

DIVERSITY is the key to success in weight loss and maintaining fantabulous health!

So maybe you've just started training at the gym building muscle, weigh about 150 pounds, and eat around 100 grams of protein per day. On your off training days you're wise-owl smart to up your protein a touch to encourage continued muscle growth. This instigates a surplus of amino acids in your blood, favorable for lean muscle mass creation.

Even in the protein department don't be afraid to switch it up for faster results.

Fallacy Three - Your body has a limit of protein it can use in one sitting.

The Truth - Talk about a wives' tale from the olden days! Your body continuously changes the amount of protein in needs and uses on a regular basis. If you gain ten pounds of sex-pot lean muscle, your body needs more protein to sustain this muscle and build more!

With protein you're best to ensure you get a little too much for your size and health goals. Listen to your body, watch and learn, and it won't take you long to figure out how much you protein you need to build your ultimate body.

Fallacy Four - You can't use protein as an energy source.

The Truth - Where the beep did you hear that one? Now if you aren't getting enough complex carbohydrates in your diet, your body will resort to burning fat and then some muscle for energy. But by making sure you're eating enough protein for protein synthesis, your body won't break down your muscle for protein use. Just make sure you're getting enough lean protein and complex carbs in your diet, and you won't have to worry about losing muscle or not being able to use protein as an energy source.

Fallacy Five - All protein is created equal.

The Truth - *Cooking Light* nutrition experts say protein quality is dependent on its ability to provide each of the 8 essential amino acids. These are not synthesized by your body and must be provided daily through your diet.

In general, complete or high-quality protein comes from animal sources. Incomplete or poorer quality protein comes from plant sources. With a few exceptions like quinoa. The only grain that's technically a complete protein source.

Fallacy Six - Eating a high protein diet is dangerous.

The Truth - That's cow crap. There is no scientific evidence that shows eating a diet of 25-35% protein is unhealthy. The problem stems from the type of protein, how it's being cooked, and of course the health of the individual.

If you are inactive, weight 300 pounds, and eat 300 grams of high trans fat fried chicken every day, then yes, you're eating style in general is deadly!

A normal person eating a healthy lean protein amount of up to 35% per day, who's active and treating their body with respect, has nothing to worry about.

NOTE: If you are battling kidney disease, or any other serious underlying medical condition, you'll want to talk first to your doctor about how much protein you should be eating each day.

Bottom line - just use common sense!

Fallacy Six - The more protein you eat the more muscle you'll build.

The Truth - Now wouldn't that be a dream come true! If you want to build lean muscle you've got to eat a good supple of healthy lean protein, but you've also got to do resistance weight training to build your muscles.

FACT - Muscles don't just grow on trees!

Eating a healthy protein-complex carb rich snack before and after training, will encourage your body to build lean muscle and blast fat. This is assuming of course you're eating healthy to begin with.

Fallacy Seven - If you want to gain weight you have to eat oodles of protein.

The Truth - You need protein to gain muscle weight. But in order to gain weight in general, it's the total calorie intake that facilitates weight gain. You could be getting an unhealthy daily dose of 80% of your calories for simple sugar carbs.

What matters is the total number of calories you're eating each day!

I can assure you if you're eating more calories than your body requires to maintain weight, you're going to get fat!

Research says, if you eat too much protein you can actually foil your plans for gaining weight. Simply because protein naturally supports that full feeling. Which of course encourages you to eat less.

If you want to gain weight, look to eating a balanced diet of lean protein, health complex carbs, and good fat.

Fallacy Eight - When you eat protein your body can't absorb calcium.

The Truth - Your bones are always in need of repair and protein is essential to this process. As well, you need protein to build muscle. Its true protein can increase the amount of calcium your body loses. A catch-22 of sorts.

Solution - Make sure you eat a diet rich in lean protein and calcium!

My Thoughts...

You're always going to run into scenarios where the information you're getting just doesn't make sense. If your gut tells you something you hear, read or see about protein just doesn't fit, make sure you ask a professional to get to the bottom of it.

Information is only useful for you if it's correct. Your health is important. So is the information you store in your noggin to create your ultimate healthy life plan.

Final Thoughts

Protein is derived from the Greek word "protos," which means first element.

FACT - You can't live without protein.

Protein is a part of every single living cells. You need it to help repair and ensure proper function of your internal systems. For everything from thinking to running, you need protein. Your blood sugar hormone insulin, enzymes, antibodies, and muscle proteins that run your body, all need protein to function optimally.

To say protein is essential to your life is 110% correct!

This introductory guide has provided you with practical insight on what protein is and how it functions, why you need it and how you can get it, and the "big picture" role of protein and how it can better your life quality.

If you've gained just one piece of useful information from my research and writing, then I'm one jolly camper. I look forward to writing many more books geared toward helping you find your healthy, one step at a time!

Last Thoughts…

*THANK-YOU for reading my masterpiece. I hope you learned a little something, or at least got a few smiles.
*I would appreciate a millisecond or three of your time for a quick review, to help me build my masterful book empire higher.
*Whatever you do, don't forget to smile, and of course, check out my website for more of my e-Book masterpieces at: www.flawlesscreativewriting.com

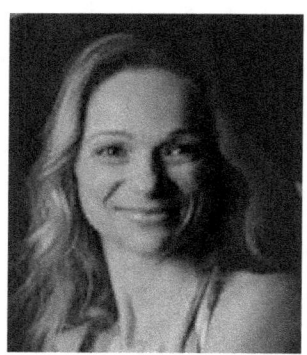

Thank you!
Cathy ☺